The quieter you are, the more you can hear.
(Chinese proverb)

For all who want to change something (to himself)

Regina Lahner

Meditation
Made Easy

With Singing Bowls

Proven Texts
Instantly and Easily Applicable
For Individual- and Group-Work

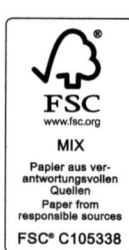

Cover design: Friedrich G. M. Roedig, Vallendar

Resources: Own & stock.xchng® vi www.sxc.hu

Image of Regina Lahner: Robert Graf

Lectorates: Senta Konopke and Anna Lahner

Translator: Dr. Georg Woodman

Bibliographic Information: Deutsche Nationalbibliothek
Original edition: German

ISBN: 978-3-8423-4517-1

1. Edition in English 2016   © 2016 Regina Lahner

Production & publication: BOD Books on Demand GmbH, Norderstedt

About the author: Regina Lahner was born in 1965 in Mönchengladbach/Germany. She's been living since her age of 2 in Bavaria/Germany and occupied herself early on in life with natural healing and all health-related topics. In 2000 she underwent an education-program of 1 year as a Dr. Edward Bach Flower Essence Remedies Therapist, and later on worked independently in the field of advice, education and seminars, and since 2005 she's offered a distant-study program of 10 months to become a Dr. Bach Flower Essence Remedies Therapist. In the same year she accomplished her education „Tibetan Sound-Bowl-Massage" at the Sebastian-Kneipp-School in Bad Wörishofen. As a referent and seminar-chair in the field of Dr. Bach Flower Essence Remedies (speeches/workshops) and singing-bowls (courses, workshops, meditation, and creational sound-painting) Mrs. Lahner is active at numerous public schools in South-Bavaria. For some years now Mrs. Lahner teaches interested persons through intensive-seminars to become Singing-Bowl Sound-Massagists.

Detailed information can be retrieved via www.bluetenberatung.de and www.tibetische-klangschalen-massage.de

Table of Contents

Preface   8

Why even Meditation?   10

Fundamentals and Directions   12

Preparation of Meditation   15

Ending of Meditation   20

Seasons and inner Harmony   22

Easiness and Relaxation   29

Clarity and Decision   33

Energy and Powerplace   36

Tranquility and Harmony   43

Sound, Color and Healing   47

Breathe yourself free   56

Woman - Meditation   59

Sakura - Meditation   65

Mediterranean Journey of Senses   69

Journey of Senses to Tuscany   74

South Sea Meditation   78

Journey through the Provence   81

Mallorcan Almond Blossom   84

Journey through the Galaxy   89

Shooting Star Meditation   95

The Power of the Moon   99

QR Code for more Information   104

Preface

After my first book „Sound Massage With Singing Bowls Easy Done" calls and emails from interested readers, students or course-practitioner reach me who have learnt and participated in meditation.

Examples:
"I've gotten an offer to conduct a course. Could you render some concrete tips how to add a sense-journey afterwards, or a meditation with Singing Bowls?"

Or:
"I'd urgently need a meditation-text for my students (kindergarten-kids, clients, patients, home-inhabitants, etc.). Can you help me?"

And:
"My children are oftentimes restless, so, what Singing Bowl phantasy-journey could I conduct with them?"

This all has compelled me to compose the nicest and prettiest texts compiled into a book.
I now wish you lots of fun in trying, converting and using the texts applied.

Notice:
You certainly may use all my materials in private sector of application, however, I'd like to ask you, if or when used in commercial application do refer to me as the original author of the ideas.

In case of using any printed materials of mine I'd ask to inquire for a prior authorization for such. (Copyright!)

Why even Meditation ever in the first Place?

One appointment chases the other, and we're rushing through the day, week, month, and the year.

In daily life as well as at our jobs, it's pretty much always the same:
1000 things must be organized and done, smoothly, and we've got to function every day, standing our man, eh, woman. Oftentimes there's no time for taking a breather. And then, even on weekends, things which have been put aside have now to be done. And, ergo, there's no time remaining for recharging our drained batteries.

But then - at last: vacation, holidays!!

Would be nice, wouldn't it? The stress still goes one when packing (have I got everything?), then at arrival, the weather at location, the accommodation, the food, the kids, the partner...

Does that not all sound just too familiar?

In our constantly in hectic increasing world is it now not even more inclining important to retrieve some placidity back into your life, and create some oasis for tranquility and relaxation?

But I already hear some objections...

"Well, I've got some much, up to my ears. And there then I'm supposed to take some time out?! Just to lie down there?! And do nothing?"

Yep, exactly!
- Take a break here and there, brief, but do it.
- Pause briefly ever now and then.
- Set a clear Stop!
- "Carpe diem", cease the moment!
- Become attentive again.
- Become tranquil from the inside.

...and then being able performing better again!

"Well, yeah, that sounds about right. But, HOW do I achieve that?"

Regretfully, no panacea-solution for that.
The methods to find to one's inner balance differ as multitude as there are people.

For one there's sport,
for another a walk into the steam-room,
and yet for another a retreat into a corner steeped into a book,
or,
one then does try meditation after all.

Important though, one must take the time for it!

Fundamentals and Directions:

There's nothing esoteric about meditation, though.
To me it just an simply means to take a brief break from daily life, to be by oneself, and to have spirit, body and soul come to rest, so to regain needed energy for the daily drudgery.

Especially the stressed person has initially issues with relaxing.
Thoughts keep drifting off, to one's unattended errands, or one's imagination is too impaired to undergo meditation.

Here the sonorous sounds of the Singing Bowls can do wonders. Subconsciously they remind us on our time in mother's womb, as we conceived the impacts in a dull sound and in floating conditions.

Even if one just concentrates simply on the sound of the bowls one enters soon a relaxed constitution, which then soon disallows any disturbing thoughts to emerge. In case the Singing Bowls are placed rather near the meditating person the vibrations might be even felt through the underpad one's lying on.

In a meditation-case solely with Singing Bowls it's quite helpful to have 5 different bowls available. But, I suggest so, the sounds of these bowls must be in harmony to one and the other. Sizes of the bowls are not relevant, though.

I recommend to use at least 3 bowls, 2 matching darker sounds, synonymous to one's heartbeat, and a middle-tone, that would be quite pleasant and 1 lighter one for the 'wake-up'.

In case you plan to arrange both massage and meditation at one then it's certainly better when the bowls are selected based on size, sound and weight as well.

In the massage it depends much on the to massaging person's bodyweight which seized bowls to be used:

300-500g = (small heart-bowl, light sound) for the upper body-region and the 'wake-up'.

500-900g = (large heart-bowl, still light sound) for the upper body-region.

900-1100g = (joint- or also universal bowl, medium sound) with a large sound-spectrum and for the joints.

1500-2500g = (small pelvis-bowl, dark sound) for the back- and stomach-region.

2500-3500g = (large pelvis-bowl, very dark sound) as above.

If the practicer performs the meditation in a small group, the skilled person can place a bowl directly onto a person and strike it there.

Tip:
All bowls ought to be struck outside at the upper section below the rim, softly and gently. Use your sentimental touch for that.

Attention - Important:
Don't render any soundbowl-massage to a pregnant person, and also don't receive one in case of pregnancy!

Chronically ill or persons with i.e. a pacemaker, remaining surgical screws or plates, cancer-sufferer, or persons with any other form of illness ought to consult an MD or practitioner prior.

If you plan to place the bowls directly onto the participants then you must select bowl-size according to the person's body-weight.

This book is complete, complex and close to the practical application of such Singing Bowl massage, and it can be administered without any further pre-knowledge.

If you'd desire more info or practical knowledge for such sound bowl-massage I refer to my initial book "Sound Massage With Singing Bowls Made Easy".

Preparation of Meditation

You'd need, depending on application, several felt-clappers or -bobbins, matching the sizes of the bowls and, at least 1 but better even 3 bowls, which are harmonized to each other.

In case you're in a larger room or one with poor acoustics, a larger wooden mallet could do better; and as an underlay for the bowls a camping- or yoga-mat would do just great.

All participants should wear loosely fitting clothes, and then make it themselves comfy, either on a chair or directly on the floor, with a cushion or soft pad. Such session could easily be conducted outdoors during summertime, but it's recommended having a blanket ready if it'd cool down.

The ones assumed position should be maintained during the entire session.

The best time is either in the morning, to gain placidity for the day ahead, or, evenings, to reach gentle relaxation for the night.

Tip:
Suiting the theme or daytime you may apply scents and fragrances. For that you may use some drops of 100% high-quality etheric oils for each participants on

a cloth or cotton-ball. This then may be placed upon one's body or near the nose.

Routine-suggestion:
Briefly introduce yourself to the participants. This produces a relationship of trust and a pleasant basis.

Tell a short tale of the idea and concept of those sound-bowls, i.e.

"These sound-bowls, I name them Singing Bowls, derived from the eastern countries India, Nepal and Tibet and are being known there for thousands of years. Originally, however, they were simple cooking dishes. Some time ago, one accidentally hit one of those bowls and experienced a quite pleasant sound. Over time then the manufacturing and the alloys had been modified in that way that they served greatly for religious rituals.

In the middle of the 80is, a German named Peter Hess visited India, and he encountered the idea of using sound and especially the vibration of those bowls
to transmit over onto human bodies, hence human bodies are made up to 75% of water, causing the inner self of one to swing harmoniously. In the meditation with these Singing Bowls, nevertheless, it's not primarily about the vibrations caused but primarily the soothing sounds and the positive effect upon the sub-consciousness."

Ask around initially if any person has had any previous experience with the bowls, or a meditation of any kind. Accordingly, further conduct ought to be

16

continued. It's quite logical and sensible to especially meditation-novices to approach gingerly. And for that there are several techniques of use:

From the outer to the inner recognition:

For example, you may strike one of the bowls and ask the participants to close their eyes. Through the conscious and focused listening to the sounds and the ultimately petering one's senses for the

- inner self,
- bodily sensitivities,
- own thoughts,
- own breathing rhythm

are being steered towards.

Via active contraction and relaxation of the muscles you can direct the meditating persons to concentrate on their inner selves.

Tip:

The higher goal in meditation is to perceive everything just observant not judging. Don't react to outer impulses, focus absolutely onto your very self.

The exemplary introductions of meditations may certainly be varied upon gusto.

Please do explain though to beginners the procedures of a meditation, which could look like this:

- no speaking during meditation
- maintain one's assumed position with-out changing
- no one may be disturbed during meditation
- in case one is attacked by coughing should quietly leave the room
- prior to the session one should visit the bathroom (toilet)

Advise your participants that you'd address them in the lesser formal way by their first names to gain closer access to one's inner. Just saying so that nobody gets the impression I wouldn't know social etiquettes.

You can explain to a novice prior that it'd be perfectly normal if he/she had initially a hard time to relax and focus. In case it'd be a reoccurring problem he/she could attempt focusing on one's own breathing-rhythm and the sounds.

Then wish everyone a great time in relaxation, and begin reading your pre-arranged texts.

Important practical note:
In the following texts I've been using blanklines, to prepare you to pause accordingly. A larger distance indicates a larger break in reading, naturally.

In case you'd not be able to sense lengths of breaks repeat the read text once or twice in your mind. That usually suffices to give the participants enough time visualizing your words spoken. During the reading break you're welcome to strike the bowls.

Let them sound off long enough, but do not allow them to fade out into silence.

Ending of Meditation:

The longer a journey or meditation takes place, the more often it happens that participants fall into a trance-like state and some even fall completely asleep. Therefore, it is to assure that participants "return" with their senses and mind completely into the reality, especially important for those who'd be driving a vehicle back home.

I usually use a method to 'wake-up' the participants, i.e. I'm counting to 5 to indicate the conclusion of the journey.

I request that everyone activates and contracts the muscles, and moves about. That way one is guided from the state of relaxation back into reality's drudgery.

Once all have opened their eyes again I always use a bright-sounding bowl I'd strike 3 times with increasing intensity and using hereby a smaller wooden mallet.

Attention:
This bright sound could easily
perceived shrill and unpleasant, so proceed this way only when ending a meditation/journey.

It'd be fine if you ask each one of the meditators afterwards about their experience and feelings. But I suggest doing so only in smaller groups; a larger group would just burst the time allotted for.

That way you'll gain experience for your further sessions to come, enabling to improvements.

But enough of the theory now, let's jump into practical application now.

Seasons and Inner Harmony

We start with a sound-meditation which addresses the seasons. It'll give you during the course more and more inner rest and harmony. For a deeper approach into yourself I'll address you in the casual and familiar way by your first names, if you'd not mind.

Now, lie or sit, most comfortably, though, in any way you desire.

Close your eyes.

Check with your closed eyes if you're in the comfiest position.

Perhaps some adjustment in your posture?

Make it yourself really comfortable.

Pay now attention to the sounds surrounding you coming from the bowls I'm going to strike.

Also watch your thoughts still rushing through your head.

Feel now how all that becomes indifferent to you.

You know now there's nothing you're forced to do or perform.

You just lie or sit there, completely relaxing and carefree.

Everything around you becomes meaningless.

Feel you feet, how and where they maintain contact to your surface.

Feel now how your calves relax.

Also, your thighs getting heavier and more relaxed.

Then go up your spine in your imagination.

Start at your back, and slowly move up.

You feel your thoracic and cervical spine.

Enjoying now the sounds of the bowls guiding your imagination.

Take your time for those thoughts.

Then you wander to your head in your imagination.

Check whether your facial muscles are perfectly relaxed.

Check your eyes.

Are your lids slightly shut, or are the pressed closed?

Feel how and where your tongue is in your mouth.

Your breathing is of fine rhythm and goes in and out.

It's perfectly relaxed and quiet with your breathing.

Now travel in your imagination to your arms.

Feel how they become pleasantly heavy, warm and loose.

Both arms are perfectly heavy and warm.
Pleasantly warm.

You're now quite relaxed and tranquil.

Enjoy this state of tranquility as intensely as possible, and let the harmonious sounds take effect upon you.

If there still a thought, well, just send it away on one of those white little clouds.

Now, just imagine, it's become spring.

Can you smell the fresh, clean air surrounding you?

It all smells so intensely, especially today.

There on the meadow grows yellow dandelion.

Perhaps you see the first buds in the twigs of the trees?

Listen to the chirping of the birds!

They're happy over the warming sun-rays after the long winter.

Feel how spring is, and breathe it deep in, deep in.

And now, imagine, summer begins, slowly...

You're passing by over a beautifully blooming stretch of grass.

The air smells sweet and fragrant.

Do you discern the scent?

Look at the countless flowers growing here.
They shine in many bright and intense colors
and ways.

Do you hear the buzzing of the bees, the chirping of the grasshoppers?

A small glittering creek provides you fresh and clean water.

You're perfectly relaxed and tranquil, and you enjoy the sunrays on your skin.

Our journey through the seasons goes on, and we're approaching autumn now.

You're again strolling...

Take a look at the colored leaves on the trees!

A sudden gust whirls the leaves off the ground into the air.

You look after them, and then you discover some migrating birds in the sky.

Do you hear their quiet calls?
In front of you are some berry-bushes with sweet fruits on.

Perhaps you'd like to taste some?

You enjoy their flavor, and you just feel great!
We slowly now move toward our last station, and it's becoming winter.

The sky is clear and blue.

It's snowing, and a snowflakes lands right onto your nose.

You feel how it slowly melts away.

The air is cold, but you're dressed warm and protected.

The snow beneath your feet is soft and tender like cotton.

The trees are coated in a fine rime.

And it glitters from everywhere like countless gems.

Can you smell the clear snow-air?

Do you feel how the air penetrates into your lungs, and how your head and your thoughts getting clearer and cleaner?

Take now all these positive feelings and sounds of inner happiness and tranquility deep into yourself.

Take them into your day-by-day drudgery, and recall of them every time you'd feel like.

Any time you may enter this state, whenever you feel like.

We're about concluding our journey through the year in the following order and fashion:

Keep your eyes still closed.

Move your hands now vigorously, and make them to fists.

Take a very deeeeeeeeep breath, and begin to stretch and stretch again.

Now, also move your arms and legs.

With every breath you now take you're becoming more and more awake.

I'll count to 5.
At 5 you're opening your eyes, and you're completely relaxed and feel just great.

1
2
3
4
5

Now you're awake.

Return to this room, into the now and here.......

Become aware of where you are at.

Perhaps you'd like to linger for a short while in the same position, there, where your journey had begun?

Easiness and Relaxation

We now come to a sound-meditation, rendering you easiness and relaxation.
I'll, as usual in meditation-sessions, address you by your first names to penetrate your sub-conscience deeper.

Please, close your eyes now.

Sit or lie as most comfortably as possible on your underpaddings.

Trace your breathing for just a moment.

You can feel how your breathing goes,
in and out,
in and out,
in and out...

That way you're becoming more and more relaxed and tranquil.

Your belly raises and sinks, automatically, with every breath you take, and there's nothing you'd have to do about it.

Up and down,
up and down,
up and down.

Your breathing is regular and calIt breathes you.

29

Now imagine you're lying down on a wonderful, green meadow.

Now see and smell the fragrance of the scenting flowers, and above blue and clear sky.

You sense the openness and tranquility.

Hither and there appears a small white cloud.

If there're emerging unnecessary thoughts in your head, just let them come, and go.

Just like the little cloud comes, and goes.

You become lighter and lighter.

Your body transforms,
you become a feather.
You are now a feather, tender and soft.
Look at yourself now,
how you look, what color you have.

Are you a tiny, or a large feather?

Are you soft and fleecy,
or rather firm and solid?

And now a gentle breeze picks you up,
carries you up higher and higher,
as much as you please.
Take a closer look up there,

what is all you see?

Feel how it is being lifted up,
becoming weightless,
being carried by the air.

And feel how the wind carries you on,
farther and farther away.

Enjoy this feeling of lightness and freedom!

Unleash your fantasy, and listen to the pleasant
sounds that accompany you.
Absorb these sounds and feelings deep into yourself.

You always may recall upon them anytime you feel
like under stress.

Call them up at your own gusto.

Enjoy this feeling just for another moment longer,
and then arrive back onto the ground.

Return back to your own image.

You are you again.

Begin to stretch yourself, and take a deep inhale.

Stretch yourself like a cat would.

Open your eyes.

Yes.
You've returned to the room.

You are relaxed indeed, and you feel comfortable and quite well.

Trace your sentiments for another moment or so.

If you'd like we can talk about your experience...

Clarity and Decision

In this sound-meditation which deals with the topic clarity and decision you might receive an answer on the problem that has you currently preoccupied.

I, as usual, will address you by your first names.

You now sit or lie comfily on your underpad.

You've shut your eyes, and feel relaxed and calm.

You feel comfortable, and you're anticipating the soothing sounds to come, which will guide you deeper and deeper into your inner balance.

We're in a garden now, and you've that feeling as if time has ceased to exist.

Tranquility and joy reign in this garden here.

You feel pleasantly warm and the sun feels wonderful on your skin.
You stroll along a path, leading you to a beautiful round meadow.

And in its middle there's a great lake.

At its shore there's a nice bench, inviting you to linger for a while.

See how calm and quite the water's surface is, not a breeze moves the mirror-like lake.

It's exactly like a glittering mirror.

Thrilled as you are, you're looking into it.
What can you see there?

Perhaps some person you'd like asking something?

Or, does there emerge a question where you'd like having an answer for?

Perhaps you're at a point of making a decision, and now seeking an option?

You've got now all the time in the world seeking for answers or obtain clarity.
Your thought flow unrestricted and unrestrained by the various sounds of the Singing Bowls.

Engage yourself, and let things flow freely.

Listen to your gut's-feeling and your inner voice.
Perhaps it now wants to tell you something...

Have you already found an answer?

Then slowly distance yourself from the images before your eyes.

Perhaps you might need to repeat this meditation a few more times at home to obtain the desired clarity and results.

Any time you feel like, you may bring yourself back into this constitution of meditation.

But now ready yourself to end this exercise soon.

Conclude the exercise in the following manner, but keep your eyes still closed, though.
Vigorously move your hands, clinch them to fists.

Stretch yourself.

Strongly move your arms and legs now.

Thereby breathe deeply in and out.

Now you'll breathe, in and out,
deeply...
Deep, in- and out,
breathe...

And in conclusion, open your eyes again.

Become aware where you are at, in which room.

And, if you like, you may tell your experience.

Energy and Powerplace

This Singing Bowl massage is about the topic of energy; you'll be here led to a place where you may return in your mind any time during your hectic day-by-day routines.

I'll address you, as typical in meditation-sessions, by your first names, allowing me to deeper penetrate into your inner self.

Make it yourself as comfy as you will, either on a chair, or directly on the floor.

You now shall feel the heaviness of your body, and you feel quite warm and pleasant.

How do you sit/lie on your surface?

Are you really comfortable?

Do you have established contact to your matting you're on?

Which parts does your body rest on?
You feel your breathing how it smoothly goes in and out.

Go with your attention once again into your entire body.

Visualize how you sink deeper and deeper onto the underpad with every breath you take.

You feel your heart how it beats evenly and quietly in rhythm.

In case your eyes are still open, close them now, or in a few minutes.

Perhaps you already feel how you sink deeper and deeper into relaxation with every tone...

...and how your legs becoming heavier and heavier.

Your arms rest heavily next to your body.

Your head too doesn't need to carry all the weight any longer, and it can let go and relax.

Begin to relax your forehead now.

You feel a refreshing, cooling scent of fresh peppermint on your forehead.

You feel your eyelids relaxing, your mouth's corners dropping.

Your facial features become quite soft and gentle.

If there're still some thoughts on your mind, just let them flow away, as a dropping leave from a tree onto the creek's waters.

You can feel how the relaxation continues throughout
your whole body.

With each and every sound of the bowls and with
each exhale you feel your body drifting into looseness
and relaxation.

Your neck, your shoulders,
relax - your shoulders which have burdened
some load in your life.

Your back turns warm and cozy.

With every exhale you relax more and sink ever
deeper into your underpadding.
Perhaps you feel the warmth in you already, or, in a
few seconds.

You feel how the warmth spreads throughout your
body.

In your neck,
shoulders,
your back - and you've that pleasant scent of
peppermint in your nose, on your forehead.

Your breathing-rhythm eases more and more, and
you feel being carried out from this room by the
harmonious sounds of the bowls.

They carry you to a very special location; a place where only you have access to, and a place that renders you tranquility and calm and power as well.

It could be a place you already know, perhaps from your last vacation?

Perhaps that particular location becomes existing just in your mind.

It may be a place high up in the mountains, within the woods, or by a lake?

It's all just so as you desire, as it is just for you.

Look around in the landscape, in which you're at now.

Look at the heavenly sky, its beautiful color!

Look at Mother Nature, with all her plants, flowers, and animals.

Feel the warm air on your skin, sense it fragrant aroma.

Feel the ground beneath your feet, enjoy your emotions and sentiments you're now just having.

And now, stroll a few steps in your mind...

Gradually you discern something in the near distance: it's becoming clearer.

It could be a cave, an igloo, a house - something just catering to your wishes, and that's where you now just want to be.

It's your personal power-place, your resting and your retreat.

And now look around even closer.

What do you recognize?

Enter, and feel the atmosphere, the mood, coming from this place.

Listen to the sounds that now surround you.

Is it bright or dark in this room?

How are the walls, how's the flooring?

Are there any things? A bed, a chair?

You've the chance now to furniture your room at your very gusto.

You may change its color, its fitting, its light - just the way you desire.

You're now perfectly relaxed and calm.

You feel quite well in your personal room now.

And now, feel deep into yourself.

Feel the happiness, the contentment, the power
within you, which just in this moment you realize so
much.

Enjoy the individual sounds of each Singing Bowl.

Let all you thoughts simply flow,
you just feel so protected and free!

Let your feelings just come and go -
just be yourself.

With every sound-off of the bowls
your energy keeps increasing.

Refuel yourself with this soundfull energy,
take the energy now deliberately into yourself.

But now it's the time where we'd have to
depart from our power-place.

You feel re-energized, strong, and refreshed,
and recharged with power!

You now can master you daily drudgery easily and
without any problems.

Return now slowly back.

To the room where your journey began.

Let your breathing become deeper and more intense
now.

Inhale fresh air with each breath you take.

Begin to stretch yourself.

Open your eyes now:
1
2
3
4
5

You're now fully awake,
and you've returned into the here and now.

Trace after your emotions for a short while.

And,
if you feel like it, you may talk about it afterwards.

Tell us how it had looked, at your power-place!

Tranquility and Harmony

We begin now with a sound-meditation which shall render you over its course serenity and harmony.

I'll address you, as standard in meditation, by your first names,

Simply to penetrate deeper into your inner self.

Lie or sit most comfortably, on the floor, or a chair.

And close your eyes now.

Perhaps you'd want to adjust your position somewhat?

Make it as comfy as possible.

Now listen to the chirping of the birds,

And the harmonious sound of the Tibetan Singing Bowls

Which shall embrace you in just a moment.

Feel how all your thoughts become indifferent now.

Everything around you becomes indifferent now.

You just lie there, completely and perfectly relaxed.

Feel your legs how they've got contact to your underlay.

Now slowly proceed up your spine in your imagination.

Begin at the pelvic region, and move upward.

You feel cervical- and thorax-spine,

while you enjoy the sounds of the bowls   ,
following alongside.

Take your time in that thought.

Then, in your imagination, you go up into your head.

Check if your facial muscles are completely relaxed.

Check your eyes, your forehead…..

Are your eyes shut tight or loosely closed?

Your breathing goes easy, you in- and exhale softly,
gently.

Your breathing is perfectly calm and evenly.

Now follow to your arms in your imagination.

Feel how they're comfortably warm and heavy.

Both arms are loose and relaxed,

warm and heavy.

You are perfectly calm and relaxed.

Enjoy this condition of tranquility and relaxation

as intensely as possible.

Let the sounds take effect on you.

In case there's some thought left,

send it on a journey on a small white cloud.

We're now in an enchanted forest

and you've the feeling as if time has stopped to exist.

You feel pleasantly warm

and there's a soft breeze blowing over your skin.

You stroll along a narrow path

leading you soon onto round meadow.

In its midst there's a small lake

and alongside the shore a bench,

Inviting you to sit down and linger.

You'll now take in the sounds of the Singing Bowls,

feeling the silence and nature's sounds,

emanating from this place.

And now you ready yourself, slowly, leaving this place.

I now may ask you to please return into the here and now.

Conclude the meditation in the following fashion:

Keep the eyes still closed.

Move your hands vigorously and clinch fists.

Now stretch out.

Move hands and arms now harshly......

...and breathe deep in and out.

Now you'll breathe deep in and out, please.

Finally, you open your eyes now, and –

you're back, becoming aware where you are at.

Sound, Color and Healing

Most people have certain physical incongruities and disharmonies, which become apparent during the day-by-day routines.

Naming one would be the tension-headache, accompanied usually with some milder back-aches.

Perhaps one feels just too overburdened.

Specifically for that condition I've got here for you the meditation, titled "healing".

You'll again be addressed by your first names.

Once again you desire to drift off into relaxation with the harmonious sounds of the Singing Bowls.

For that you'll now close your eyes.

Breathe deep and evenly.

In and out,

in and out,

in and out.

Everything around you becomes meaningless.

Everything that burdens you vanishes before your inner eye.

With every breath you take you become more and more placid.

Your body becomes quite heavy.

You sit or lie perfectly relaxed on you cushioning surface.

In distance you discern the sounds of the Singing Bowls.

You're at a wonderful garden now.

The air is fresh and clean, your lungs open widely, just to intake this precious element into yourself.

Clean air flows deep into your lungs' branches, fueling you with energy.

You deeply exhale the used-up air, allowing refuel with fresh energizing air.

You feel much better already, since you can so consciously in- and exhale.

In and out,

in and out,

in and out...

With that deep breathing and the harmonious sounds,
oxygen flows into you and revives your spirits.

Adrenaline rushes through your veins and you'd love
jumping up in excitement!

But are you actually ready for that?

I think your body needs somewhat more time....

You lie down on a patch of green lush grass.

The grass carries you like a soft cushion, and you feel
like floating above the ground.

Continue to breathe deep in and out, feel the intaking
air cleaning and strengthening your body.

Later you'll imagine a variety of colors which shall
penetrate into you and begin healing your body.

Now, surround yourself with the color "Blue".

You see this 'blue' like through a fog, embracing you, shrouding you completely in.

This 'blue' now touches every organ in you, flushes every cell.

Take your time, feel how this 'blue' spreads completely throughout, fulfilling you perfectly and absolutely.

Everywhere where healing is required 'blue' flows over there just by itself.

Next now you imagine the color "Green".

This 'green' surrounds you and fills you into its shroud.

Give your organism the time to absorb this 'green' and let it have taking effect.

You've got sufficient time, all the time you'll need.

Inhale the healing 'green' into your body.

You feel how your vitality becomes stronger and now feel your blood-circulation, too.

Perhaps it feels somewhat sluggish?

Now go into your heart, and quite consciously feel your pulse, and now let "Red" fill in your entire heart, let flow a beaming 'red' throughout your body.

Lighten up all areas that would need fresh energy.

See how this 'red' now flows through your network of veins and arteries and how it fills with new life.

How it unclogs the blood-vessels and how it makes them free and transparent again.

This 'red' cleanses you and strengthens your whole organism.

It reaches every corner in your body and every even ever so the smallest fiber.

Now bestow your heart with a soft "Pink",

So it can freely and unselfishly love.

Feel how this 'pink' embraces your heart and fills the rest of your body.

See how your heart widens, how it opens up like a rose itself affecting in itself quite perfectly.

Your heart now is full of love and wonderfully pleasant feelings.

You're not just having those sentiments for others, but also for yourself.

And now, pleasantly bright "Yellow" radiates into your head-region.

Go with that through all parts of your brain, feel how each part of it is flooded by the sun-rays of 'yellow'.

The golden-yellow light chases off all negative thoughts from your sub-conscience.

Take yourself all the time with cleaning your thoughts.

You feel how more and more clarity spreads out and all negativity yields and vanishes.

The 'yellow'-light can now spread in you more and more unrestricted in you.

Your body now is cleansed, and you know, a positive regeneration-process has just kicked in you.

You're now ready taking in "White" light –

let therefore the 'white' flow in through and enjoy the color flowing in you.

It shrouds you from outside like stardust.

This color now spreads in you like a constant stream,

beginning at your toes, and exiting at your hair-tips.

You feel the color everywhere, and you feel absolutely great and in your own midst.

Now you're ready for the supreme color of all spiritual colors:

"Purple".

First, 'purple' spreads in you in a bright color in you.

Then it begins to turn darker, livelier and more radiant.

You reflect this color from the inside outward.

You feel the complete satisfaction, tranquility and the inner balance reigning in you.

Soon the time shall come where you will depart from your darling garden and where you must return into the here and now.

If you'd like, reflect upon those colors once more in order they appeared and flooded through you.

First the color of the healing blue,

then the regenerating green,

the energy-rich red,

the lovely pink,

then the beaming yellow,

the cleansing white,

and – the spiritual purple.

All the colors remain conserved in your body.

You'll take them with you, in you day-by-day, in your life.

You can recall of them any time you desire, any time you feel it's needed.

I now slowly start counting backwards from 5 to 1.

At 1 you'll open your eyes, move your arms and legs and you'll have arrived back into this room again.

5

4

3

2

1

I welcome you back into our midst.

Breathe yourself free

I welcome you cordially and look forward to the next minutes with you.

To gain deeper access to your inner self, I'm addressing you by your first names.

We now want to start our day with a relaxing breathing exercise.

For that please lie or sit down most comfily.

Close your eyes now and focus on your inner self.

Feel now how your body becomes heavier.

Your legs become heavy.

Your arms becoming heavier, more and more.

With every breath your relaxation increases.

And now – pay great attention to your breathing: how it slowly comes, and goes.

Your breathing comes and goes –
in your own rhythm.

Soft, evenly,
light and calm.

You now just breathe soft and gently,
tracing after your own breath.

Oxygen enters through your nose or mouth,
widens your abdomen
and flows into your chest-cavity.

When exhaling air leaves its way in opposite order:
First from your chest,
and through your abdomen.

You breathe in gently:
into the abdomen,
then into the chest.

You breathe out gently:
from the chest,
from the abdomen.

In: into the abdomen,
into the chest-cavity.

Out: Out from the chest,
out from the abdomen.

In: into the abdomen,
into the chest-cavity.

Out: Out from the chest,
out from the abdomen.

Please, breathe a few more times that way,

in your own speed and pace.

Now you send your breathing to a part,
a part which may cause you problems.

Try now guiding your breath exactly there,
gently,
softly.

In case there are no blockages right now, well, just
breathe to an area that seems to be important for you.

Now imagine that with every breath you take new
energy flows to that region.

And simultaneously with every exhale the blockages,
the stress,
the inner tension subside more and more.

Breathe energy in, and all burdening out.
Breathe energy in, and all burdening out.
Breathe energy in, and all burdening out.
Breathe energy in, and all burdening out.

Breathe further in and out at your own pace.

You feel more and more easiness and energy in you.

Return slowly back to the here and now.

Now you may embrace the new day with recharged
energy and fresh vitality.

Women - Meditation

This sound-meditation shall give you new energy and vitality.

I'll address you, as typical in meditation, by your first names.

Make it as comfy as you will on your surface.

You'll now feel the heaviness of your body, and you feel pleasantly warm and cozy.

How do you sit or lie on your matting?

Is it just the way you like?

Where does your body contact on the surface?

You feel your breath how it slowly enters and leaves.

It flows gently through your windpipe,
into your lower abdomen-region,
into your upper abdomen-region.

And – ultimately, into your chest cavity.

When exhaling the breath flows gently
first from your chest-room
into the upper abdomen-area,
and then from the lower belly-region out.

You're breathing at your own pace,
in and out,
in and out
in and out…

Go with your attention now deeper into your body,
and visualize how you're sinking,
deeper and deeper with each and every breath,
onto your padding.

You feel your heart,
beating in an even rhythm,
quietly,
calmly.

In case you haven't closed your eyes, please,
do it now,
or in a few minutes, though.

Perhaps you feel already how you sink deeper with
every tone,
into the relaxation –
and how your legs becoming ever heavier.

Your arms are resting heavily but loosely next to your
body.

Your head as well doesn't need to carry all its weight
any longer; it can just relax and let go.

Begin now to relax your forehead.

You feel your eyelids loosening.

Your mouth loosens, too.

Your facial features become soft and perfectly relaxed.

You can feel how the relaxation proceeds through your body.

With each sound and each breath your body loosens and relaxes more,
and deeper,
and more…

Your neck-muscles relax.

Then your shoulder-belt.

Your shoulders which have carried some burden already.

Your back becomes warm and cozy.

With every exhale you can let yourself drop,
and sink deeper into your padding beneath you.

Perhaps you feel the warmth?
Now?
Or in a short while, though.

You feel the warmth spreading throughout your body,
more and more…
in your neck,
shoulders,
back.

Your breathing becomes even calmer,
and now feel deep into yourself.

Feel the happiness,
the content,
but especially the power in you.

The power which makes you aware in just that
moment:
You are a strong woman!

You've done and accomplished quite a lot in your life,
and you're taking the other hurdle, too.

It becomes reality what you've planned.
Feel now your femininity,
your gentle side,
which may coexist with your power-side.

Feel the love you can perceive for others.

But also perceive the love you can feel for a very
special human being:
Namely yourself!

Enjoy now the various sounds of the Singing Bowls.

Let all your thoughts simply flow...

Let your feelings come and go,
let just be yourself.

With every tone of the bowls your energy and
becomes greater, and so your joie de vivre.

Fuel yourself now with that sonorous energy!

Take this energy now consciously into yourself.

Let it radiate in you,
as if it was the (spring)-sun,
warming you,
charging you with energy and power.

You feel strong and refreshed, and recharged with
power!

Now you can master your day-drudgery without any
problems.

Return now slowly back to the room,
there where your journey began.

Let your breathing now become more intensive and
deeper.

Take with each breath fresh air into your lungs.

Stretch yourself!

Open your eyes.
1
2
3
4
5

You're now quite awake and have returned into the
here and now.

Trace your sentiments for a while...

Sakura - Meditation

We stroll in our minds into a Japanese Zen-garden.

You're walking placidly over a white pebble-stone
path,
alongside of bonsais,
conifers and maple trees.

After a while you approach a crescent-shaped bridge.

If there's something that still burdens you, leave this
thoughts far behind.

Leave them behind that bridge.

And – when mentally ready - cross this bridge now.

Now there are no disturbing thoughts left.

Now take a closer look around you in this garden.

What all can you recognize?

The diverse plants and their colors and shapes are
clearly discernible.

You discover to you completely unknown plants and
flowers, partly quite exotic looking.

Now you can sense a very pleasant fragrance.

You want to know where it's coming from.

Your sight fans over the landscape.

In the distance you see a tree in full bloom.

It's a beautiful, large cherry-tree.

You approach that tree, pick one of the cherry blossoms, and gingerly pluck it off.

Now you sit or lie comfortably in the tree's shadow.

Take now a closer look at your blossom.

What color is it?

What shape are its petals?

Are they pointy or round?

How is it surface?

Is it rather smooth or rough?

How's the blossom's center?

Take a deep breath now and take in its pleasant fragrance.

You now sink with every breath you take in deeper and deeper into a cozy and relaxing condition.

You enjoy the tranquility in yourself.

You're simply yourself now.

With every exhale your inner self becomes lighter and more carefree.

You're shrouded in a wonderful room of scent, sound and color.

You amalgamate with the sound, building a unit with it.

I leave you in this dreamy world for a while...

Slowly it's time that we return back into reality.

Give your garden a farewell, and thank your cherry-flower for all that it had given and shown you.

With the subsiding sounds your thoughts return back to this place.

When soon a bright sound chimes you'll be back in the here and now.

You stretch yourself, and you breathe deeply and firmly the surrounding air into you.

Now, you'll slowly open your eyes.

Mediterranean Journey of Senses

I sincerely welcome you and look forward to the next ½ hour where you let your body, soul and spirit come to rest a little.

In the constantly increasing hectic of our world it becomes more and more important building an oasis of rest and relaxation for oneself.

I'm going to let sound different Singing Bowls during our meditation for you.

Simply try to let the different sounds take an effect on you, and just follow the meditation, so let go of any disturbing thoughts, please.

Especially initially it could happen that this won't work right off the bat, though.
If there are any thoughts going through your head, focus on your breathing and try to find back to yourself.

I wish you a wonderful relaxation.

To gain better access to your mind I'll address you by your firstnames, as so typical in meditation.

While you seeking for a comfy position your mind slowly comes to rest, too.

Take a deep breath now.

While exhaling let all burden drop,
leave your everyday-life behind,
and let everything just go.

With every inhale you take also "calm" in and with
every exhale you put out "tension".

You take in "calm" and put out "tension".

You take in "calm" and put out "tension".

You'll soon feel to desire falling deeper into this
pleasant condition of calm and relaxation.

And while you're listening to me you can send your
thoughts on to a journey.

Imagine now you're at a wonderful place, somewhere
at the Mediterranean Sea.

It's a warm summerday,
the sun is bright,
and you saunter through alleys and streets of this
idyllic fishermen-village.

You now look in contemplation at those houses with
colorful doors and either half-open or shut windows.

In front of these houses you see the typical
Mediterranean flowers and scenting herbaceous plants
planted in heavy Terracotta pots.

Before one of those houses is an elderly woman
sitting beneath a blue sun-umbrella,
crocheting a white doily.

There in front of her stands a basket,
full of fresh and juicy fruits.

The elderly nods friendly at you, hands you one of
these fruits.

It's your favorite fruit!

You thank that lady,
and you bite into the fruit - and you just enjoy it!

I'm now asking myself if you even could taste the fine
aroma of that fruit on your tongue.

Full of energy you run down through those narrow
alleys, and you enjoy the slightly salty wind from the
sea and the coolness reflecting from the houses.

From far you discern sounds of a church-bell and
something that reminds you of a market.

Curiously you walk an, and you discover booths and
stands with clothing,

food,
and household goods.

You approach the scene, and you observe the hustle
and bustle.

When you've seen enough you continue your stroll
through the village.

The path leads you passing a fountain-well.

Perhaps you'd like to refresh yourself a little and drink
some of the delicious water?

Can you feel how fresh and clean it tastes?

Can you feel how the cooling water pleases on your
skin?

Replenished and full of energy you begin your return-
trip back through the little Mediterranean village.

Slowly it's time getting your attention back to the here
and now.

I'll count to 5 for that purpose:

1 – your breathing becomes more conscious now.

2 – you take a deep breath.

3 – you slowly move yourself.

4 – your movements become more intensive, you contract your muscles.

5 – you open your eyes, and you have completely returned into the present.

I hope this meditation was able addressing all of your senses and it has been a pleasant experience for you.

Thank you very much!

Journey of Senses to Tuscany

I welcome you to our 20-minute meditation session of relaxation.

Please try to visualize everything I'm saying during our meditation and absorb the impressions non-judgemental.

If there should occur disturbing sounds or thoughts just let them come, and go again.

Concentrate again onto yourself and the sounds of the Singing Bowls.

I'm going to address you by your firstnames, that way gaining deeper access to your sub-conscience.

This is a journey for all your 5 senses,
which will bring you into the Tuscany, Italy.

Concentrate onto your own breathing rhythm and close your eyes now.

Make it yourself comfy on your mat and listen into yourself for a brief moment.

Our journey begins in the tranquil city of Florence.

We stroll together over the weekly market.

Take a look at the many booths, filled with fresh fruits, veggies and many other sweets and goodies.

If you like you can sample some of it all.

Perhaps you van even taste it on your tongue?

Somewhat farther down you discover a stand with the typical herbs of the region.

The aromas and senses flatter your nose, and they make you feel so placidly relaxed.

They let forget all tension and worries of your daily life.

Breathe these fragrances deeply in and out.
In and out…

With every breath you take more and more placidity spreads out in you.

You feel how you come more and more to rest.

You sink deeper and deeper into relaxation.

Since you're being that relaxed now you like taking a closer look of Tuscany.

You mount a horse-drawn coach, which soon will bring you into the hinterland.

Here grow left and right of the road typical cypresses, vineyards, and olive-trees.

In the far you see elegant looking houses in white and yellow.

It's a pretty summer-day, a soft breeze goes.

The sun warms you.

I am wondering if you actually could even feel the warmth and the wind on your skin.

You now intensively enjoy the moment of your wonderful holiday and the special magic of this rolling hill landscape.

The soft snorting and rhythmic hoof-beats of the horses let you even deeper sink into relaxation.

You can take in the whole positive feeling of the tranquility and relaxation deep into yourself.

You can recall of it later on any time you feel, any time whenever you see pictures of the Tuscany, or something else reminds you of Italy.

You now may dream a little and have some time for you sentiments to enjoy.

And just like any and every holiday, this day too reaches its end soon.

With the romantic impressions of the setting sun behind those hills – it's about time...

...time for finding back into the here and now.

1 – perceive your breathing now more consciously.

2 – contract tour muscles slightly.

3 – let your breathing-rhythm become more intensive.

4 – begin slightly to move your body, the stretch yourself.

5 – and, if you feel willing now, open your eyes again.

I hope you could enjoy your journey for your senses:

the hearing,
the feeling,
the smelling,
the touching,
the tasting...

South Sea Meditation

I welcome you to the journey for your senses.

To gain better access to you I'll address you by your firstnames, as typical in meditation.

Just imagine, you're traveling on a beautiful summer-day on your dream-cruiseship, towards the South-Sea.

The water is calm, and it glitters in countless tones of blue.

The ship anchors before a small island, and there you disembark.

In the distance you hear the gentle chirping of exotic birds.

You roam a bit, enjoying the fresh seabreeze.

You feel the soft sand beneath your bare feet.

Once you strolled around enough
you seek a shaded place beneath a palmtree,
and there you make it yourself quite comfortable.

Breathe in once, very consciously.

The sweet scent of to you unknown flowers reaches deep down into your lung-branches, filling you with happiness and a feeling of good fortune.

You even begin to smile a bit.

You now feel quite intensely your inner center.

Your stability within yourself, growing with each and every exhale.

I leave you alone with your relaxation and rest to enjoy so for a moment just by yourself.

The desire in you awakes to take a closer look of the island before returning back to the ship.

Now you get up in your mind, and you find a narrow pathway, leading you onto the middle of the island.

Left and right of the way line up some exotic plants with ripe fruits like bananas, mangoes, pineapples, and papayas.

You select a specially ripe and juicy fruit, and you just enjoy it!

Can you even taste the aromatic flavor in your mouth?

Full of energy and refreshed you start your return to

the ships mooring-place, which will bring you back to your initial location where you started off on your journey.

I'll now count to 5.

1 – you begin to breathe deeper and more intense.

2 – you move yourself slightly.

3 – you clinch your hands to fists.

4 – you stretch yourself.

5 – you now open your eyes, and you're back to the here and the now.

I hope you were able to have your soul and spirit let dangle during your journey to the South Sea and replenish your energy for your daily life.

Much thank for your interest.

Journey through the Provence

Our (scent)-journey begins in France's South-East, in Grasse.

In this small but world-famous town are from selected ingredients those extracted essences being used to create the aromatic perfumes for the entire world.

From there we drive further up into The Provence, to the well-known lavender fields.

Make yourself as comfortable as possible on your mat.

Perhaps you'd like to adjust your position somewhat?

It's a pleasantly warm summer-day.

Already from far distance you can see, as far as the eye can reach, the violet fields of blooming lavender.

Also in the air already, even though still in greater distance the fragrance is perceivable, the fine and relaxing scent.

The lavender works calming on your spirit and now, with every breath you take, you'll sink deeper and deeper into your undermat.

The more you approach the fields, the more calm and placidity amplify in you.

All tension and stress of daily life, all thoughts that roam through your head – it all dissolves by the fragrant aroma of the lavender.

And with exactly that help of the lavender-fragrance you now sink deeper and deeper into a relaxing condition.

The color violet stands for soul-balance.

It also has a cleansing and pain-alleviating effect on your body.

Imagine now, with your next inhale you'll take a bright violet into yourself.

Imagine now how this violet imbues your body, that way triggering the self-healing mechanism in you.

Now let flow that violet to a part of your body which now needs relaxation or healing.

With every breath now that violet becomes darker and the effects of that color even intensify.

And now, every time you see the color violet you'll feel calm and your self-healing powers are being activated again.

Slowly now it's time to return into our reality, though.

You clinch your hands into fists.

You take a deep breath.

You slightly move your whole body now.

You stretch yourself.

You open your eyes.

I hope you were able to turn yourself off during our meditational journey into the Provence and were able to truly enjoy it intensely.

Majorcan Almond Blossom

I'd like to take you now onto a little journey in fantasy, to Spain, to Island of Mallorca.

Engage yourself to that journey, relax your body, mind, spirit for the next 15 minutes…

To obtain better access to your inner self, please allow me to address you by your firstnames, as it so is typical in meditation-sessions.

I wish you a great relaxation.

Try now for the next several takes of breath to feel consciously your breathing going in and out.

Your breath flows in, gently and easy, and out again…

in… and again out… and

in… and out again.

Now imagine spring has just arrived.
On the island of Mallorca the almond-trees are in bloom now.

It's a warm spring-day und you feel pleasantly warm.

The sunrays warm your whole body.

They warm first your hands, then your feet.

You can feel that way that you're sinking deeper and deeper into pleasant relaxation caused by the warmth.

The entire island is by the millions of blooming blossoms dipped into a sea of white and pink.

The fine, sweet scent of the blooms impregnates the air.

You stroll through the picturesque landscape a little.

After you've strolled along for a while you get the desire to rest beneath those shade-spending almond-trees.

There's a mighty one which grants to the soothing shade.

You rest at its bark, and you feel the power radiating from the tree into you.

It is a quite old tree, its roots penetrate deep into the soil, and it had mastered some storms in its life.

You can feel how this tree now renders some of its power, to you, the power you'll need for the daily struggles of yours.

You feel you've reached the center of yourself now.

You feel now relaxation and placidity sprawling out more and more within you.

The beguiling, sweet scent of the almond-blossom lets you come to rest more and more.

Perhaps you can even sense the aroma in your nose now?

You look up to the sky, and you see some small clouds passing by.

If there're arising some thoughts in your mind, well, send them on one of those clouds onto a journey.

That way nothing can disturb your relaxation.

In distance you hear some seagulls crying, while a gentle wind blows over from the sea to you.

I'm wondering if you might even taste the slightly salty air from the sea on your tongue?

After you've rested sufficiently you get up again.

You're now walking bare-feet over the soft grounds and you're recharged with fresh energy.

Meanwhile you let roam your view into the far distance and over the sea.

In the distance you discern some boats, looking to you almost like toys from far up here.

Absorb now all these feelings of calmness, freedom and placidity deep into you.

You may, in future, any time you desire, teleport yourself in your mind back to this location, which renders you so much rest and relaxation.

But soon the time has come to bit farewell to Mallorca and the almond-trees.

I'll now count from 5 to 1:

5 – Take a deep breath now.

4 – Your breathing becomes more intensive now and adapts to your normal breathing.

3 – You do some easy movements, and have them becomemore intensive.

2 – You contract, from the bottom upward, your muscles.

1 – Open your eyes.

I hope you could enjoy intensely your time out for relaxation and rest.

In the next days, if so needed, simply try to recall your meditation, if you are in a stress situation.

I wish you lots of fun and success with that!

Journey through the Galaxy

I cordially welcome you and look forward to the next 30 minutes of rest and relaxation with you.

I will then also appeal to the familiar way by using your first names to get a deeper access to your heart.

We now start right from the comfort of our chair or our cushion of a journey through our galaxy.

I wish you a lot of fun and a nice relaxation.

Your body is now completely relaxed on your padding... and then, if you're willing, please close your eyes.

Mentally we float now surely toward the heights towards the Sun.

You can feel Sun's rays warm your skin now.

The closer we travel towards Sun, the more pleasant you feel the warmth on your skin.

On our journey into space, we first meet our good old Moon with its bright, by craters covered, silvery translucent surface.

You can now feel the dynamics and power of Moon executing so intensively on Earth, and at the very same moment on you.

Fill your entire body with this strength, or send them to a place in you where it might just cause problems and new vitality there's in need.

You look briefly back onto our Blue Planet with the huge oceans and continents and gladden yourself at this breathtaking sight.

Maybe there even flits now a smile on your face and you can enjoy the beauty of this sight so really intense deep down in you.

Our journey is coming to the 2nd planet of the Solar System, namely... Venus.

The Evening and Morning Star, which deep at night isn't visible, shines in reddish-white mist that looks quite impenetrable.

The Venus is considered Goddess of Life and renders you now new vitality.

We then fly totally relaxed toward our next planet, Mercury.

It is a brownish and very small planet circling in Solar System directly from the Sun.

He is according to Roman mythology the messenger of the gods and in astrology the planet of communication and understanding.

Now we orbit our great soothing Sun.

Sun, our Mother of Planets, stands for vitality and gives you now the necessary heat, power and strength that you need for your life.

In a big crescent now we cross again the orbital of Mercury, Venus, back, passing Earth, in the direction of Mars, our neighboring Red Planet, the first of the outer planets.

Mars spends you now new determination and willpower.

We move on through the asteroid belt to Jupiter, the largest planet in our Solar System.

Jupiter stands for happiness and success and provides always new confidence in your life when something just doesn't work out once in a time.

Finally we reach Saturn, the second largest of our planets, with its humongous rings surrounding. Saturn is already an unimaginable 1.2 billion kilometers away from us.

Saturn gives you the necessary stamina and discipline that you need in all your projects.

We float on to the bluish Uranus; with its power it supports you for all new ventures and all new beginnings.

The blue translucent Neptune stands for humanity and idealism and it always grants you new feelings of harmony and hope.

We have now arrived on our trip through the galaxy at the last of the planets in our Solar System, the outermost and smallest planet of all, Pluto.

In times when you may already think of giving up,
Pluto gives you in all aspects and life-areas always new
motivation.

But soon our journey through space is coming to an
end, and we slowly flying back to Earth.

Mentally we go again by all the outer planets:
small Pluto,
blue Neptune,
bluish Uranus,
then gigantic Saturn with its huge rings,
then great Jupiter, and...
the Red Planet, Mars,

until we're full of new energy, vitality, and beautiful
feelings return to Earth again safe and sound.

Our breathing becomes faster again, we stretch our
arms and legs.

I'm going to count backwards from 5 to 1:
5
4
3
2
1

We now slowly open our eyes, and are back in the
here and now...

Shooting Star – Meditation

I cordially welcome you tonight to our Shooting Star Meditation and wish you a nice relaxation.

You may wish upon something also, which might even come true in the course of meditation; who knows!?

To get a better access to your sub-consciousness, I will, in meditation so typical, address you by your firstnames.

If your thoughts meanwhile in-between should digress briefly, try to concentrate again on your breathing, thereby finding easier back into meditation.

I now wish you a nice relaxation!

Now steer your attention consciously on your own breathing-rhythm.

Feel how the breath gently flows in your body, and how it flows out again.

Your breath flows entirely in your own pace quietly into your body,
in…
and it flows gently out.

And now take a deep breath with which you can easily relinquish all worries and tension of everyday life.

You are now only you and you need not to worry about anything else.

The vibrations and sounds of the Singing Bowls are spreading now very slowly and very comfortable in your body and you are sinking deeper and deeper into a state of harmony.

Imagine now, you're lying at dusk in a beautiful meadow at a lake.

You're enjoying the last warm rays of a hot summer day on your skin.

Gradually it is pleasantly cool and soon breaks in darkness.

Countless stars appear sparkling and radiant in the firmament and are reflected in the water.

You start a little dreaming and let this stunning impression penetrate deep in you.

Suddenly you discover a shooting star.

You are very happy and you're allowed to wish upon something.

Watch the shooting star, until it is no longer visible.

And now you again are thinking of very personal wish.

Imagine now again exactly again what it feels like for you what has now changed in you.

I wonder what happens when your wish is being fulfilled soon.

You have the next few minutes enough time to all imagine it exactly and to dream a little.

Gradually, however, turn the thoughts back to reality.

For that you take a deep breath now.

Start moving easily.

Let your movements and breaths become more intensively.

And if you then are willing you may open your eyes again!

I hope you were able to relax pretty well?

I would like to express now to our fingers crossed that your wish may come true soon and everything is exactly how you have imagined it.

The Power of the Moon

I am glad that you want to relax for the next 20 minutes with me with a Moon-meditation.

I'll address you by your firstname in order to reach your sub-consciousness at a deeper level.

Before we begin you should find a comfortable position, while I would like to mention some things worth knowing about our earth satellite to you:

The Moon orbits in a cycle of 28 days the Earth, influences by its gravitation the tide... and also the living beings on our planet Earth.

The Moon is very well visible by the remote of 384,400 km to us without any aids with our naked eye and is so far the only celestial body that has already been entered by people.

The Moon is said to have certain powers that supposedly even affect our lives.

These forces are now accompany you through meditation...

Now check again your posture and your position on your underpadding.

Do you lie you really comfortable?

Now close your eyes and heed only on your breathing.

All thoughts and sounds around you are now becoming more and more indifferent.

You lie just there, completely relaxed.

Your breath flows entirely in your own pace quiet in and out your body...

in and out...

in and out...

in and out...

We now go mentally through the 28-day continuing lunar cycle and begin at the full moon.

And now imagine, you'll be illuminated by the full moon.

You might even see his friendly moon face, do you?

Its rays fall like the warm sun light quite pleasant to your body and gently shroud you.

You feel the peace and secureness of the mysterious-looking light that now illuminates you and the whole surrounding.

I wonder if you can perhaps feel the strong force of renewal and the zest of Full-moon even in you?

What do you implicitly still want to do in your life?

Take this energy of the Full- moon now deep in to you and fill your body, or a place in your body, with it.

You can now let go of old things and open up for a new beginning.

Immediately after the Full-moon, the phase of the Waning-moon starts.

Imagine, as the Moon slowly decreases more and more... its sickle narrows more and more.

Everything is now lighter and more jauntily, all you do succeeds just like by itself.

The force of the Waning-moon makes energy flow again in you, and a cleaning and renewal process kicks in.

Take this energy now on in you and try to send it to a place in your body that just needs cleaning and renewal.

Now the Moon is barely visible, New-moon is imminent.

This lunar energy helps to you a fresh start, and new ideas or projects are just waiting to be soon implemented.

What did you want to do for some time?

Which plan or idea you'd still need support?

Imagine now a bit of what you'd achieve or do/want in the future and how the New-Moon supports with all its might in and for that future.

The Moon-cycle is nearing its end, 21 days have passed since Full-moon and the Moon continues to increase.

The self-healing powers are stimulated, everything is geared to development, inclusion and growth.

Even your ideas and plans still can continue to grow.

In this powerful phase can mature your projects; and might they be implemented already in your plan step by step?

Imagine it again once exactly...

If you cannot succeed within one Moon-, then

there're still indeed many more cycles and options available.

The cycle of the moon is approaching its end.

28 days have passed and we now mentally again have arrived at Full-moon.

You can at any time in the future, if you need support in your life, recall again upon the power of this meditation.

And now let the bright light that still encases you, slowly darken.

Come with your thoughts back to reality.

Clinch your fists,

take a deep breath, start to move,

and stretch yourself,

and then re-open your eyes.

I wish you much joy and fun with the meditations.

Do you own a Smartphone?

Do you own a smartphone? About this QR-Code you can get more information:

Homepage
Singing-Bowls

Homepage
Dr. Edward Bach Flower Essence Remedies

Twitter
News

Facebook: "Bachblüten Klangschalen"

Ich bedanke mich von Herzen bei meinem Mann Peter, der mich ermutigt hat dieses Büchlein zu schreiben und der mir mit Rat und Tat zur Seite stand. Ohne Dich wäre das Buch wahrscheinlich nie in Druck gegangen.

Auch bedanke ich mich herzlich bei meiner Schwester Eva, die ebenfalls Korrektur gelesen und mir manchen wertvollen Tipp gegeben hat.

Last but not least möchte ich Ewa Staudigl für die interessanten Stunden danken. Unsere Treffen haben mich zu Silvers Abenteuern inspiriert.